CONTENTS

BEST MOTIVATIONAL BOOK EVER: <u>RISE UP SOLDIER</u>

COPYRIGHT

DEDICATION

This book is dedicated to those who have grown tired of being left behind. To the ones who are ready to adopt a soldier mindset and conquer their fears. To those who refuse to settle for a mediocre life and instead strive for greatness in all areas of their lives, this book is for you. It is for the dreamers, the doers, and the ones who believe that success is achievable for anyone who is willing to work hard and persevere through obstacles. To my family, friends, and loved ones who have supported me throughout this journey, thank you. This book would not have been possible without your unwavering encouragement and belief in me. Finally, to those who have been searching for a roadmap to success, I dedicate this book to you. May it serve as a beacon of hope and a reminder that with the right mindset and tools, anything is possible.

INTRODUCTION

Welcome, soldier, to the "Best Motivational Book Ever : Rise up Soldier." This book is not about visualizing nor dreaming, but rather about taking concrete steps to help you become a soldier in life. It's about developing the discipline, focus, and determination that you need to overcome any obstacle and achieve your goals. Inside these pages, you'll find practical strategies that will help you unleash the warrior within and fight for your dreams like never before. You'll learn how to develop a warrior mindset, build a strong foundation, set goals that will inspire you to take action, overcome obstacles, and embrace failure as a stepping stone towards success. In the part 10 of this book, you'll be inspired with powerful speeches of a motivational speaker who understands the challenges that you're facing and knows how to help. The given speeches will encourage you to keep fighting for your dreams, even when the going gets tough. "Best Motivational Book Ever : Rise up Soldier" is more than just a book, it's a roadmap to success that will guide you through the ups and downs of life and help you become the warrior you were meant to be. If you're ready to unleash the warrior within and rise up to your fullest potential, this roadmap to success is for you. It will equip you with the tools, knowledge, and inspiration that you need to conquer any challenge and achieve your biggest dreams. It's time to unleash the soldier within and start living your best life.

PART I - FROM CIVILIAN TO SOLDIER

The civilian mindset may sometimes be characterized by a lack of discipline, focus, and purpose. Individuals in civilian life may not always have a clear sense of direction or mission, and may become easily distracted by trivial matters, potentially lacking the drive and determination needed to achieve their objectives. "From civilian to soldier" is a term that refers to a transformation that goes beyond just wearing a uniform and carrying a weapon; it requires a shift in mentality, meaning : applying the same principles of military strategy and mindset to your everyday life. This transition is not only essential for those who choose to serve in the army but can also have positive impacts on those who adopt a soldier's mindset in their daily lives. Soldiers are renowned for their discipline, focus, and purpose. They possess an obvious sense of mission and value teamwork, discipline, and sacrifice. Embracing a soldier's mentality can help you develop these qualities and achieve success in various areas of life. It requires a commitment to hard work, determination, and a willingness to overcome obstacles. If you're ready to make the transition from civilian to soldier, you must be prepared to follow orders and rise up to the challenge. The key is to embrace the mindset of a soldier and apply it to your everyday life. "From Civilian To Soldier" is not just a phrase but a call to action, urging you to take control of your life, set clear goals, and work tirelessly to achieve them. Are you ready to embrace the soldier's mentality and rise up to the challenge?

SECTION I : EMBRACING THE SOLDIER'S MENTALITY

A warrior mentality is a force to be reckoned with, it is the ultimate mindset for achieving success in all areas of life. It requires strength, discipline, perseverance, and a strong sense of purpose. When you embody a warrior mentality, you become a focused, confident, and determined individual who refuses to back down in the face of adversity. No matter how tough the road ahead may seem, you possess the motivation and drive to keep pushing forward. The warrior mentality is all about taking risks and facing challenges. It's about recognizing that the path to success is often paved with obstacles and setbacks, when you embrace this mindset, you empower yourself to achieve personal growth and development that goes beyond what you ever thought possible. It's time to adopt the warrior mentality and let go of any self- doubt and fear of failure. Embrace the fact that challenges and difficulties are a natural part of life, but remember : you have the strength and resilience to overcome them. By pushing beyond your limits and stepping outside of your comfort zone, you will achieve greatness. Just like soldiers who train to push themselves physically and mentally, you too must be willing to push yourself beyond what you think is possible, you need to rise up. Embrace challenges that seem impossible, face your fears, and push through obstacles to achieve your goals because you develop the mental and emotional toughness needed to overcome any obstacle that comes your way. You must unleash your inner warrior and achieve the success you deserve. With the warrior mentality, anything is possible.

First Mindset : Avoid Self-Doubts

Self-doubt is an inherent facet of the human experience, and it can manifest in multifarious ways, including apprehension of failure, dread of rejection, or uncertainty of one's capabilities. For soldiers, who are frequently confronted with high-stakes situations demanding unwavering performance, conquering self-doubt is imperative. Through rigorous training and unwavering resolve, soldiers have honed techniques to combat self-doubt that can be effectively employed by civilians in their everyday lives. Here, we will explore how soldiers combat self-doubt and provide practical strategies that civilians can adopt to overcome it as well.

1-Adopt A Growth Mindset

Soldiers possess an incredible trait that sets them apart from the rest: a growth mindset. It's the unwavering belief that with hard work and practice, they can develop their skills and abilities to become the best version of themselves. This mentality enables them to overcome the toughest of challenges and rise above self-doubt. You don't need to wear a uniform to adopt this mindset! Whether you're a student, a professional, or a stay-at-home parent, you too can embrace the growth mindset. By viewing obstacles as opportunities to learn and grow, you can boost your confidence and overcome any self-doubt that may be holding you back. Don't be afraid to take challenges as great opportunities to push yourself to new heights. With a growth mindset, you can unlock your true potential and achieve greatness.

2-Seek Support

Soldiers know the importance of having a strong team by their side. They lean on each other for motivation and support, knowing that together they can achieve greatness. And just like our brave servicemen and women, you too must seek out the support of your loved ones and mentors when you face moments of self-doubt. By opening up and sharing your fears, you will gain a fresh perspective and receive the boost of encouragement that can help you overcome any obstacle. Seek out those who can lift you up and watch as you soar to new heights.

Second Mindset : Push Beyond Your Limits

Soldiers embody the unwavering spirit of determination, perseverance, and resilience. They know no bounds and refuse to back down in the face of adversity. Whether it's battling physical challenges, conquering mental barriers, or facing combat, soldiers exemplify the true meaning of pushing beyond limits. You too can harness the power of determination to push yourself further than you ever thought possible. It takes practice, courage, and an unwavering belief in yourself, but the results are worth it. From now on, don't settle for mediocrity even when the going gets tough. Embrace the soldier's mindset and push yourself to achieve greatness. "The only limits that exist are the ones you create in your mind."

1-Physical

One of the key techniques used by soldiers to push beyond their limits is physical conditioning. Soldiers are required to maintain a high level of physical fitness to perform their duties effectively. They are trained to push themselves beyond their limits so as to improve their physical abilities. You can also benefit from physical conditioning by setting fitness goals, gradually increasing your physical activity, and pushing yourself to improve your physical abilities.

2-Breaking Tasks Down Into Manageable

You have the power to conquer any challenge, just like our brave soldiers. The secret lies in breaking down your goals into smaller, manageable steps. By taking things one step at a time, you can focus on making real progress towards your dreams and stay motivated throughout the journey. Don't let the enormity of a task hold you back. Break it down and show yourself what you're capable of.

3-Use Teamwork

Soldiers also use teamwork to push beyond their limits. By working together as a team, soldiers can support and motivate each other and achieve their objectives more effectively. We can also use teamwork to push beyond our limits by working with others towards shared goals, and by seeking support and motivation from others. Soldiers are trained to embrace discomfort as a normal part of the training process. By pushing themselves beyond their comfort zones, soldiers are able to improve their physical and mental abilities. You can also benefit from this mindset by embracing discomfort as a normal part of the growth process. By pushing yourself beyond your comfort zone, you can improve our skills, abilities, and resilience. Soldiers push beyond their limits by using specific techniques and strategies, such as physical conditioning, breaking tasks down into smaller steps, teamwork, and embracing discomfort. You can also use these techniques to push beyond your own limits and achieve your personal and professional goals. By using these techniques and cultivating a resilient mindset, you can push beyond your limits and achieve success.

SECTION 11 : THINK AND ACT LIKE A SOLDIER TO SUCCEED

Soldiers are trained to think and act in a specific way, they are taught to be disciplined, focused, decisive, and trained to work as a team and to prioritize the mission above all else. These traits are not just valuable in the military, they are valuable in all areas of life. If you want to succeed in life, you must adopt a military mindset. You must learn to be disciplined, focused, and decisive. You must learn to work as a team and to prioritize your goals above all else. When you have the mindset of a soldier, you are better equipped to overcome challenges and to achieve your objectives. To think like a soldier, you must let go of self-doubt and fear of failure, take ownership of your life and your goals, be willing to push beyond your limits, and find your purpose and motivation by doing specific things.

One Of The Most Important Qualities You Must Have Is :

Discipline :

Soldiers are taught to follow orders and to stick to a routine. They are trained to be mentally prepared for any situation. This discipline helps them to stay focused and to accomplish their goals. In the civilian world, discipline is just as important. You must be disciplined in your work, your relationships, and your personal life. Without discipline, you are likely to procrastinate, to make poor decisions, and to fall short of your goals.

Focus:

Soldiers are trained to keep their attention on the mission at hand. They are taught to ignore distractions and to stay focused on their objectives. This focus helps them to avoid mistakes and to accomplish their goals quickly and efficiently. In your daily life, focus is equally important. You must stay focused on your goals, even when you're faced with distractions and obstacles. You must learn to ignore the noise around you and to keep your eyes on the prize.

Decisiveness:

It is another critical trait of the military mindset. Soldiers are trained to make quick and effective decisions, even under pressure. They are taught to weigh the risks and benefits of each option and to choose the course of action that is most likely to achieve their objectives. Being decisive is also crucial, you must be able to make quick decisions and take action when necessary. You must be willing to take risks and make tough choices, even when the outcome is uncertain. Thinking and acting like a soldier can help you achieve success in all areas of life. By developing discipline, focus, and decisiveness, you will surely overcome challenges, achieve your goals, and become the best version of yourself. Rise to the challenge, respect these steps and embrace the warrior within you.

PART II - THE BATTLEFIELD OF LIFE

Welcome back to the Best Motivational Book Ever : Rise Up Soldier. In this chapter, we will be delving into the challenges that soldiers face on the battlefield. We'll explore the enemies that you'll encounter, both within and without, and provide you with the tools and strategies you need to overcome them. First, let's talk about the enemies within. These enemies are fear and doubt. These enemies can undermine your confidence and prevent you from achieving your full potential. Next, we'll turn our attention to the enemies without: the obstacles, criticism, and naysayers that you'll encounter on your journey to success. We'll show you how to stay focused on your mission, and come out on top. Soldier, Gear up and get ready to conquer your ennemies.

SECTION I : THE ENEMY WITHIN

The enemies within are surely the most insidious and dangerous of all. These enemies take the form of fear and doubt. Fear tells you that you're not good enough, that you don't have what it takes to succeed. Doubt whispers in your ear, sowing seeds of uncertainty and causing you to question your abilities leading you to undermine your own efforts and sabotage your own success.

How Do You Overcome These Enemies?

The first step is to recognize that they exist, and that they are not the truth. Fear, doubt, are simply thoughts and emotions that you experience, but they are not the reality of who you truly are or what you can achieve. You must learn to separate yourself from these negative thoughts and emotions, and to see them for what they really are: temporary obstacles that will be overcome.

Mindfulness:

One powerful way to combat these enemies within is through the practice of mindfulness. Mindfulness is the art of being present in the moment, fully engaged in the "here and now". It is a way of observing your thoughts, emotions without getting caught up in them, and of cultivating a sense of inner peace and clarity. By practicing mindfulness, you can learn to quiet the negative voices in your head, and focus your attention on the present moment.

Positive Sel-Talk:

Another powerful tool for overcoming these enemies within is the practice of positive self-talk. This means consciously choosing to speak to yourself in a positive, empowering way, rather than allowing negative self-talk to dominate your thoughts. Instead of saying "I can not win against them" try saying "I know who I am, I will win no matter what" By choosing to focus on your strengths and your potential, you will build your confidence and overcome doubts and fears.

Resilience and determination:

Ultimately, the key to overcoming the enemies within is to cultivate a mindset of resilience and determination. Recognize that setbacks and obstacles are a natural part of the journey, and that every failure is an opportunity to learn and grow. Remember that success is not a destination, but a journey, and that every step you take towards your goals is a victory in itself. With the right mindset and tools at your disposal, you can overcome the enemies within.

SECTION I I : THE ENEMY WITHOUT, HOW TO DEAL WITH CRITICISM, NAYSAYERS

In this section, we'll focus on the other sort of enemies, those outside of you - the ones that come in form of criticism and naysayers.

Criticism :

When you're on a mission to achieve greatness, you can expect that there will be people who will criticize you. They may not understand your vision, they may not believe in your abilities, or they may simply be jealous of your success. Whatever the reason, their criticism can be a powerful force that can either discourage or motivate you. It's important to remember that criticism is not necessarily a bad thing. In fact, it can be a valuable tool for growth and improvement. If you receive constructive criticism, take it as an opportunity to learn and grow. Use it to identify your weaknesses and find ways to overcome them. But if the criticism is unwarranted or unjustified, don't let it get to you. Instead, use it as fuel to prove your critics wrong. Soldiers usually face criticism in their line of work. Whether it's from their superiors, their peers, or the general public, criticism can be difficult to handle. However, t h e y are trained to deal with criticism in a way that allows them to learn from it and use it to improve their performance. Let's explore how soldiers deal with criticism and the way you can use these techniques in real life.

Don't Take It Personally:

Soldiers are trained to view criticism as an opportunity for growth and improvement, rather than as a personal attack. They understand that criticism is often intended to help them become better at their jobs, and they try to approach it with an open mind. In real life, you can use the same technique by trying not to take criticism personally. Instead, view it as an opportunity to learn and grow.

Focus On The Message:

When soldiers receive criticism, they exhibit a unique approach that sets them apart from others. Instead of becoming defensive or argumentative, they prioritize the message itself, rather than the person delivering it. This characteristic distinguishes them as individuals who are resilient, adaptable, and committed to improvement. Soldiers are trained to value feedback as a valuable tool for growth and development. They understand that criticism is not a personal attack, but rather an opportunity to identify areas that need improvement. They actively listen to the underlying issues being raised, regardless of how the message is delivered, and make efforts to understand and address them. We can learn from this approach and apply it to our interactions with others. When receiving criticism, it's crucial to detach ourselves from any emotional response and focus on the content of the message. Rather than getting defensive or dismissive, we can choose to actively listen and understand the concerns being raised. This involves putting aside any personal biases or preconceived notions about the person delivering the criticism and instead, objectively analyzing the content of the feedback. By focusing on the message rather than the messenger, we open ourselves up to valuable insights and opportunities for self- improvement. It allows us to see beyond the delivery style or tone of the criticism and identify the underlying issues or areas that may require attention. This approach promotes a growth mindset and encourages continuous learning and improvement. By prioritizing the message, we can also build stronger relationships with others. It shows maturity and professionalism when we are willing to listen and take it in without becoming defensive. It also creates an environment of open communication, where constructive criticism is welcomed, and honest feedback can be freely given and received. Adopting a soldier-like approach to receiving criticism by focusing on the message rather than the messenger can greatly benefit you in your personal and professional lives. It promotes a mindset of continuous improvement, enhances your ability to objectively assess feedback, and fosters positive relationships with others. So let us strive to prioritize the message, and not let our emotional reactions hinder our opportunities to growth and become stronger.

-Take Actions:

The art of taking action is a fundamental trait that soldiers understand and apply in their training. They recognize that criticism, whether it comes from their commanding officers or fellow soldiers, serves as a valuable tool for growth and development. Rather than shying away from criticism or becoming defensive, soldiers are trained to embrace it as a catalyst for change. In the military, criticism is not viewed as a personal attack, but rather as an opportunity to identify areas for improvement. Soldiers are encouraged to actively seek feedback and to listen with an open mind to any critiques that are offered. They understand that ignoring criticism or responding defensively would only hinder their progress and limit their potential for growth. Taking action on criticism involves a proactive approach. Soldiers are trained to take steps to address the issues that are raised, rather than dwelling on the negativity or shifting blame. They take ownership of their mistakes or shortcomings and view them as opportunities to learn and improve. Whether it's through additional training, practice, or seeking guidance from their superiors, soldiers take concrete actions to rectify the identified areas of concern.

Moreover, soldiers understand that taking action on criticism requires a mindset of continuous improvement. They don't view criticism as a one-time event, but rather as an ongoing process of self-assessment and self-improvement. They are constantly looking for ways to refine their skills, enhance their performance, and become more effective in their roles. They understand that complacency is not an option, and that taking action on criticism is essential for their personal and professional development. This approach can also be applied to everyday life. When faced with criticism in various aspects of life, such as at work, in relationships, or from friends and family, adopting a soldier's mindset can be beneficial. Rather than dismissing criticism or becoming defensive, one can choose to take action on it. This could involve reflecting on the feedback received, identifying areas for improvement, and taking proactive steps to make positive changes. For instance, if a colleague provides feedback on a work project that highlights areas that need improvement, instead of feeling discouraged or defensive, one can use it as an opportunity to take action. This could involve seeking additional resources or training, revisiting the project with a critical eye, and making necessary changes to enhance the quality of the work. By taking action on the feedback received, one can demonstrate a growth mindset and a willingness to learn and improve. Soldiers understand that criticism is a valuable tool for growth and development, and they are trained to take action on it. They view criticism as an opportunity to identify areas for improvement, and they proactively take steps to address the issues raised. This mindset of continuous improvement and taking ownership of one's mistakes can be applied in various aspects of life, enabling individuals to embrace criticism as a catalyst for positive change and personal growth.

-Seek Feedback:

Finally, soldiers understand the importance of seeking feedback. They actively seek out criticism and feedback from their superiors and peers, as well as from those outside of their immediate circle. They understand that feedback is essential for growth and improvement. In real life, you can use this technique by actively seeking feedback from others. Ask for input on your performance, your ideas, and your work, and use this feedback to make improvements. Soldiers have developed effective techniques for dealing with criticism that can be applied in real life. By not taking criticism personally, focusing on the message, taking action, and seeking feedback, you can turn criticism into an opportunity for growth and improvement.

-Naysayers:

These are the people who will tell you that you can't do something, that your dreams are impossible, or that you're wasting your time. Naysayers can be a major obstacle on your journey to success, but it's important to remember that their opinions don't define you. You are the only one who can decide what you're capable of achieving. When you encounter a naysayer, don't let their negativity bring you down. Instead, use it as motivation to prove them wrong. Let their doubt fuel your determination and push you even harder to achieve your goals. Dealing with naysayers can be a challenging task, especially when pursuing personal or professional goals.

Soldiers are trained to handle this situation effectively, and their techniques can be applied in real life to overcome similar challenges. Here are some of the techniques that soldiers use to deal with naysayers, and how these techniques can be applied in everyday life.

Prove Them Wrong:

Soldiers are trained to use negative comments and criticisms as motivation to prove their naysayers wrong. This is achieved by focusing on their goals and pushing themselves to achieve them, despite the obstacles in their path. In real life, individuals can use the same technique by using the negative comments of naysayers as motivation to work harder and achieve their goals. By focusing on the end result and proving their naysayers wrong, individuals can overcome the negative effects of naysayers and achieve success in their personal and professional lives.Dealing with naysayers can be a difficult task, but soldiers have developed effective techniques to handle this situation effectively. By focusing on the mission, staying positive, developing a strong support system, and using negative comments as motivation to achieve their goals, soldiers have successfully overcome the negative effects of naysayers on the battlefield.

These techniques can be applied in real life to overcome similar challenges and achieve success in personal and professional lives. As a soldier on the battlefield of life, you will face many enemies. But with the right mindset and determination, you can overcome them all. Use criticism as a tool for growth, let naysayers fuel your motivation, and find ways to overcome any obstacle that comes your way. Stay strong, soldier, and keep marching forward.

Soldiers Learn From Failure:

For soldiers, fear of failure can be a major obstacle to success. By using specific techniques, soldiers can destroy fear of failure and achieve their objectives. you can also benefit from these techniques and use them in their daily lives to overcome your fear of failure.

Mental Rehearsal:

One of the key techniques used by soldiers to overcome fear of failure is mental rehearsal. Before a mission, soldiers mentally rehearse the steps they will take and the potential challenges they may face. This helps them prepare mentally and emotionally for the mission, reducing the fear of failure. Civilians can also use mental rehearsal to prepare for challenges and overcome their fear of failure. By visualizing success and preparing for potential obstacles, individuals can build confidence and reduce their fear of failure.

GOAL-SETTING:

Goal-setting is a powerful technique utilized by soldiers to achieve success in their missions. As part of their rigorous training, soldiers are taught to set clear, measurable goals that serve as guiding principles for their actions and decisions. These goals help soldiers stay focused and motivated, even in the face of adversity, and enable them to overcome their fear of failure.

Setting clear and achievable goals is essential for soldiers, as it allows them to have a clear vision of what they want to accomplish. Whether it's capturing an enemy stronghold, completing a mission, or achieving a specific objective, soldiers are trained to establish specific, measurable, attainable, relevant, and time-bound (SMART) goals. This helps them create a roadmap for success, with each goal acting as a stepping stone towards the ultimate objective.

Moreover, goal-setting provides soldiers with a sense of purpose and direction. It helps them prioritize their efforts and resources towards the most critical tasks, ensuring that they stay on track and do not get overwhelmed by the challenges they face. Goals serve as a compass, guiding soldiers through uncertain and chaotic situations, and helping them make informed decisions to achieve their desired outcomes. In addition to providing motivation and focus, goal-setting also helps soldiers overcome their fear of failure. Soldiers operate in high-stress environments where failure can have serious consequences, both for themselves and their fellow comrades. By setting clear goals, soldiers are able to break down their missions into smaller, more manageable tasks. This allows them to approach their objectives step-by-step, reducing the risk of failure and increasing their chances of success.

Soldiers are trained to learn from setbacks and adjust their goals and strategies accordingly, rather than being deterred by failure. The benefits of goal-setting are not limited to the military realm. Civilians can also apply this technique to overcome their fear of failure and achieve success in various aspects of life. Whether it's in their personal or professional lives, setting clear and achievable goals can help individuals stay focused, motivated, and resilient, even when faced with challenge. By breaking down their larger objectives into smaller, actionable goals, individuals can create a roadmap for success, monitor their progress, and make adjustments as needed to stay on track. Goal-setting is a valuable technique used by soldiers to achieve success in their missions. It helps them stay focused, motivated, and resilient, and enables them to overcome their fear of failure. You can also benefit from this technique by setting clear, measurable, and achievable goals in various areas of your life. You can stay on track, remain motivated, and ultimately achieve their desired outcomes. We can also use goal-setting to overcome their fear of failure. By setting clear, achievable goals, individuals can stay focused and motivated, even in the face of obstacles.

Focus On The Present Moment

Another technique used by soldiers is to focus on the present moment. Soldiers are trained to focus on the task at hand, rather than worrying about the future or dwelling on past failures. By staying present in the moment, soldiers can reduce their fear off failure and stay focused on their mission.

We also benefit from this technique by practicing mindfulness and focusing on the present moment. By staying present and focused, individuals can reduce their fear of failure and make better decisions.

Embracing Failure As A Learning Opportunity:

In addition to these techniques, soldiers are also trained to embrace failure as a learning opportunity. Failure is viewed as a natural part of the learning process, and soldiers are trained to learn from their mistakes and use them to improve.

Civilians can also benefit from this mindset by embracing failure as a learning opportunity. By viewing failure as a chance to learn and grow, individuals can reduce their fear of failure and become more resilient.

Use A Team-Oriented Mindset:

Finally, soldiers use a team-oriented mindset to overcome fear of failure. Soldiers work together as a team, supporting and encouraging each other. By focusing on the mission and working together, soldiers are able to overcome their fear of failure and achieve their objectives. Civilians can also use this mindset to overcome their fear of failure. By working together with others and focusing on shared goals, individuals can reduce their fear of failure and achieve success. Soldiers are trained to overcome their fear of failure by using specific techniques and strategies, such as mental rehearsal, goal-setting, positive self-talk, focusing on the present moment, embracing failure as a learning opportunity, and using a team-oriented mindset. Civilians can also use these techniques to overcome their fear of failure and achieve their personal and professional goals. By using these techniques and cultivating a resilient mindset, individuals can overcome their fear of failure and achieve success.

PART I I I : THE SOLDIER'S PLAN

Soldiers know that victory on the battlefield requires more than just brute force. It requires strategy, planning, and a clear understanding of the enemy's weaknesses and strengths. The same is true in the battle for success. To achieve your dreams, you need a battle plan that outlines the steps you must take to achieve your objectives.

In this chapter, we will look at the essential elements of a battle plan for success. We will explore how to identify your goals, and how to create a plan that will keep you on track and motivated. We will also discuss the importance of persistence in the face of adversity. Soldiers know that battles are won not just by brute force, but by the unyielding determination to keep pushing forward, no matter how tough the fight is, if you're ready to take your dreams from the realm of fantasy to the battlefield of reality, then this chapter is for you. Let's create a battle plan together that will help you achieve victory in your personal and professional life. Remember, success is not a destination - it's a journey. And with the right battle plan and the courage of a soldier, you can conquer any obstacle and achieve any goal. Listen up, soldier, if you want to succeed in life, you need a battle plan: A plan that will help you navigate the twists and turns of the battlefield of life, and guide you towards victory. Just like in a military operation, success requires careful planning, preparation, and execution. Setting a battle plan is a critical process for soldiers in the military. It involves analyzing the situation, identifying the objectives, and developing a detailed plan of action to achieve those objectives. While battle planning may seem like a specialized skill reserved for soldiers on the battlefield, the same principles can be applied in real life to help individuals achieve their goals.

SECTION I : CONCRETE STEPS

Assessing The Situation:

Assessing the situation is a critical step in any endeavor, whether it's developing a battle plan or tackling a complex problem in the workplace. The first step in assessing the situation is to gather as much information as possible about the situation at hand. This can involve conducting research, speaking with experts in the field, and gathering data and statistics. Once you have gathered these information pieces, the next step is to analyze it in order to gain a deeper understanding of the situation. This can involve identifying patterns and trends, analyzing data and statistics, and conducting a SWOT analysis (Strengths, Weaknesses, Opportunities, and Threats). By analyzing the information in this way, you can gain a more complete picture of the situation and identify any potential risks or obstacles that may need to be addressed.

After analyzing the situation, the next step is to develop a plan of action. This plan should be tailored to the specific circumstances of the situation and should take into account any potential risks or obstacles that have been identified. The plan should also be flexible enough to adapt to changing circumstances, as unexpected challenges may arise.

One important aspect of assessing the situation is to remain objective and avoid making assumptions or jumping to conclusions. It's important to gather all available information before making any decisions or developing a plan of action. This can involve seeking out diverse perspectives and considering. Another important aspect of assessing the situation is to remain open-minded and adaptable. The situation may change rapidly, and it's important to be able to adjust your plan of action accordingly. This can involve being willing to try new approaches or pivot to a different strategy if the current plan is not working. Briefly, assessing the situation is a critical step in any endeavor. By gathering information, analyzing it, and developing a plan of action, individuals can gain a deeper understanding of the situation and identify any potential risks or obstacles that need to be addressed.Objectives provide clarity and direction, allowing individuals to focus their efforts and resources on achieving specific goals. To set objectives effectively, it is important to have a clear understanding of what you want to achieve and how you will measure success.

The first step in setting objectives is to define what you want to achieve: This involves identifying a clear outcome that you are working towards, whether it is a specific project, goal, or mission. It is important to make sure that your objective is specific, measurable, achievable, relevant, and time-bound. This means that your objective should be clear and specific, it should be measurable so that progress can be tracked, it should be achievable given your resources and abilities, it should be relevant to your overall goals and mission, and it should have a clear timeline for completion.

Once you have defined your objective, the next step is to establish metrics for success. This involves identifying specific indicators or milestones that will help you measure progress towards your objective. These metrics should be aligned with your overall objective and should be measurable, so that progress can be tracked and evaluated. It is important to establish these metrics early on in the planning process, so that you can monitor progress and make adjustments as needed. Another important aspect of setting objectives is to ensure that they are realistic and achievable. This means taking into account the resources and constraints that are available, as well as the risks and challenges that may arise. It is important to be realistic about what can be achieved within the given timeframe and resources, and to make adjustments as needed to ensure that your objectives are achievable.

Setting objectives requires a commitment to accountability and evaluation. This means regularly monitoring progress towards your objectives, evaluating the effectiveness of your strategies, and making adjustments as needed. It is important to hold yourself and others accountable for achieving objectives, and to take responsibility for any setbacks or failures that occur.

Setting objectives is a critical step in achieving success, whether in military operations or in everyday life. By defining clear objectives, establishing metrics for success, being realistic and achievable, and committing to accountability and evaluation, individuals can focus their efforts and resources on achieving their goals and moving towards success.

Executing The Plan

Executing a plan is the culmination of all the hard work that has gone into the planning process. It is the point where all the ideas, strategies, and tactics come together, and the plan is set into motion. However, executing a plan is not as simple as just following a set of steps. It requires a certain mindset, a commitment to the plan, and the ability to adapt to changing circumstances. In this section, we will discuss how to execute a plan effectively and achieve success in real-life situations.

The best thing to do when executing a plan is to have a clear understanding of the plan and the objectives that it aims to achieve. This requires a deep understanding of the plan's purpose, the strategies that will be used, and the tactics that will be employed. It is essential to have a clear vision of what success looks like and to have measurable goals that can be tracked throughout the execution process. Without a clear understanding of the plan, it is impossible to make progress towards achieving its objectives.

Another critical element of executing a plan is to have the right mindset. This involves having a positive attitude, a commitment to the plan, and a willingness to adapt to changing circumstances. It is essential to maintain a sense of motivation and focus throughout the execution process and to stay committed to the plan, even when faced with challenges and setbacks. This requires a strong sense of self-discipline and a willingness to put in the necessary effort to achieve the plan's objectives.

Besides having the right mindset, it is also essential to have effective communication channels in place to ensure that everyone involved in the execution process is on the same page. This includes clear communication of goals, objectives, and expectations, as well as regular updates on progress and any changes to the plan. Effective communication helps to ensure that everyone is working towards the same goals and that any issues or obstacles are addressed quickly and efficiently.

Adapting To Changing Circumstances:

Executing a plan also requires the ability to adapt to changing circumstances. In the military, soldiers are taught to be agile and flexible in the face of changing conditions. This same principle applies to real-life situations, where unforeseen obstacles or opportunities may arise that require a change in course.

The ability to adapt and pivot quickly is essential to achieving success in executing a plan. This requires a willingness to reassess the situation regularly, to evaluate progress and adjust the plan accordingly.

SECTION I I : THE POWER OF PERSISTENCE

The power of persistence is essential for achieving success. Just like it's essential for a soldier to stay committed to his mission, to persevere through obstacles, setbacks, to keep pushing forward no matter how difficult the terrain or the circumstances. In the same way, to achieve your dreams, you must be willing to put in the hard work, to stay focused, and to keep going even when the going gets tough. One of the key principles of persistence is the willingness to overcome obstacles. Just like a soldier who must overcome obstacles to achieve their mission, you must be willing to overcome the obstacles that stand in the way of your goals. These obstacles can take many forms, such as self-doubt, fear, lack of resources, or external challenges. But if you have the determination and persistence to overcome these obstacles, you will ultimately succeed.

Persistence requires discipline and hard work. You must be willing to put in the time and effort necessary to achieve your goals. This means sacrificing short-term pleasures and comforts for long-term success. It means being willing to work hard, even when you don't feel like it, and pushing yourself beyond your limits.The power of persistence is a key ingredient in achieving success. It requires having a clear goal, overcoming obstacles, maintaining a positive mindset, and being willing to put in the hard work and discipline necessary to achieve your dreams. Just like a soldier, you must be willing to persevere through the toughest of circumstances, to keep pushing forward, to never give up until you achieve victory.

PART IV : BUILD YOUR TEAM WORK

Soldiers, we are not alone on the battlefield of life. We have our comrades-in-arms, our brothers and sisters who fight alongside us. They are our teammates, our partners in battle, and together, we are stronger than we ever could be alone.

SECTIONI : WORK WITH OTHER SOLDIERS TO ACHIEVE YOUR GOALS

In war and in life, there is strength in numbers. No matter how skilled you are , there are limits to what you can achieve on your own. That's why it's essential to learn how to work effectively with others, to build strong relationships, and to cultivate a sense of teamwork. As a soldier, you understand the importance of working together towards a common goal. You know that everyone has a role to play, and that success depends on each member of the team doing their part.

Whether you're pursuing a career, starting a business, or working on a personal project, you need a team of people around you who can support you, encourage you, and help you achieve your objectives. But teamwork is not always easy, It requires patience, communication, and a willingness to listen to others. It also requires the ability to resolve conflicts and to work through disagreements in a constructive way. As a soldier, it's your responsibility to create an environment where everyone feels valued, respected, and heard. You need to be able to inspire and motivate your team, to set clear goals and expectations, and to hold everyone accountable for their actions. To achieve success as a team, you need to focus on creating a culture of excellence, this means setting high standards for performance and holding yourself and others to these standards. It means fostering a sense of trust and mutual respect, and celebrating the successes of your team as a whole.

SECTION I I : RESOLVING CONFLICTS AND BUILDING A WARRIORS' UNITY

As a soldier, one of the most important aspects of your role is being a team player. To achieve your goals, it is imperative that you work effectively with others. However, conflicts are inevitable in any team, and as a soldier, it's important to have the skills to resolve them effectively. Resolving conflicts requires strong leadership skills. It's important to be able to identify the root cause of the conflict and to listen to all parties involved.The best way to do it is by following these steps:

Peace Environment:

Create an environment where everyone feels comfortable expressing their opinions, you can prevent conflicts from escalating.

Common Goal:

One way to resolve conflicts is to focus on finding a common goal. As a soldier, you and your team are working towards the same mission. By reminding everyone of that mission and the importance of working together, you can help bring your team together and resolve conflicts.

Honest Communication:

Another way to resolve conflicts is to encourage open and honest communication. It's important to make it clear that all opinions are valued and that everyone has a voice. By doing so, you can create an environment where conflicts can be resolved in a healthy and constructive way. Being a successful soldier requires not only individual strength and determination, but also the ability to work effectively with others. Conflicts are bound to arise, but with the right leadership skills, they can be resolved in a way that strengthens the team and helps everyone achieve their goals. Remember, teamwork is the key to success on the battlefield.

PART V - THE SOLDIER'S CODE

The Soldier's Code means respect the three core values of a warrior, which are: honesty, integrity, and honor. These values serve as the foundation of a soldier's character and guide their actions both on and off the battlefield.

SECTION I : THE CODE'S MEANING

Honesty

Honesty is a quality that is highly valued in both personal and professional relationships. For soldiers, honesty is not just a personal attribute but a necessary component of their duty to serve their country. A soldier who values honesty will always strive to do what is right, even when it is difficult or unpopular. This commitment to honesty is rooted in the belief that it is essential for building trust, maintaining integrity, and achieving success.

One of the key aspects of honesty is being truthful with oneself. Soldiers must be self-aware and recognize their own strengths and weaknesses. This self-awareness allows soldiers to take responsibility for their actions and to make changes when necessary. It also allows them to be honest with others, as they can admit when they have made a mistake or when they need help. By being honest with oneself, soldiers can cultivate a sense of personal integrity that is essential for maintaining trust and respect. Another Important aspect of honesty is being truthful with others. Soldiers must be transparent in their communication, even when the message is difficult or uncomfortable. This requires a high level of emotional intelligence, as soldiers must be able to communicate in a way that is clear, respectful, and sensitive to the needs of others. When soldiers are honest with their fellow soldiers, their superiors, and the civilians they serve, they build trust and credibility, which is essential for achieving mission success. Admitting mistakes is a critical component of honesty. Soldiers must be able to recognize when they have made an error and take responsibility for their actions. This can be difficult, as admitting mistakes can be seen as a sign of weakness. However, by admitting mistakes, soldiers demonstrate their commitment to honesty and integrity. They also create opportunities for learning and growth, as mistakes can be used as opportunities for improvement and development. Honesty also involves being accountable for one's actions. Soldiers must be willing to accept the consequences of their actions and to take steps to rectify any mistakes they have made. This can involve apologizing to others, making amends, and taking steps to prevent similar mistakes from occurring in the future. By being accountable for their actions, soldiers demonstrate their commitment to integrity and to the values of the military. Honesty is a fundamental value for soldiers, as it is essential for building trust, maintaining integrity, and achieving mission success. Honesty requires soldiers to be truthful with themselves and with others, to admit mistakes, and to be accountable for their actions. By cultivating a commitment to honesty, soldiers can demonstrate their integrity and earn the respect and trust of their fellow soldiers, their superiors, and the civilians they serve.

Honor

Honor is a timeless concept that has been revered in human society for centuries. It represents a set of values that we hold ourselves and others to, such as honesty, integrity, and respect. In the military, honor is one of the most important values that soldiers strive to embody. A soldier who values honor will act with dignity and respect, always holding themselves to a higher standard of conduct and behavior. At its core, honor is about recognizing the intrinsic worth of oneself and others. It means valuing oneself and one's own contributions while also acknowledging the value of others and their contributions. Soldiers who value honor recognize that everyone has something to contribute, whether it's a unique skill or perspective, and they treat others with fairness and compassion. Living up to a higher standard of conduct and behavior is a hallmark of honor. It means holding oneself accountable for one's actions and taking responsibility for one's mistakes. Soldiers who value honor understand that their actions have consequences, and they strive to always act in a manner that reflects positively on themselves and their unit.

Another important aspect of honor is respect. Soldiers who value honor treat others with respect, regardless of their rank, position, or background. They understand that everyone has inherent worth and dignity, and they show respect to others by listening to them, considering their perspectives, and treating them with fairness and compassion. Honor also involves a commitment to honesty and integrity. Soldiers who value honor always tell the truth, even when it's difficult or uncomfortable. They understand that honesty is the foundation of trust, and they strive to build and maintain trust with their peers and superiors. Additionally, soldiers who value honor demonstrate integrity by doing the right thing, even when no one is watching.

Honor is a guiding principle that soldiers strive to

embody in all aspects of their lives. It represents a commitment to living up to a higher standard of conduct and behavior, and holding oneself accountable for one's actions. By valuing honor, soldiers can build trust with their peers and superiors, earn the respect of others, and uphold the values that are essential to the military and society as a whole.

Integrity

Integrity is a fundamental quality that is highly valued in all aspects of life. It is the embodiment of honesty and moral principles, and is regarded as a cornerstone of personal and professional success. For soldiers, integrity is a vital component of their identity as they are entrusted with immense responsibilities and often operate in high-stakes and high- pressure environments. The importance of integrity in the military cannot be overstated, as it is essential for maintaining trust and cohesion within the ranks, and for upholding the values and principles that the military represents. At its core, integrity is about doing the right thing, even when no one is watching. It is about having the courage and conviction to stand up for what is right, and to resist the temptation to compromise one's values or principles. This can be a challenging task, particularly in situations where there are competing interests or pressures, but soldiers who prioritize integrity understand that it is non-negotiable. They recognize that the trust and respect of their fellow soldiers, their superiors, and the public depend on their unwavering commitment to honesty and morality. For soldiers, the value of integrity extends beyond their personal beliefs and values. It is a critical aspect of their role as protectors of their country, and as representatives of the military. The public trusts soldiers to act with integrity and honor, and any breach of this trust can have serious consequences not just for the individual soldier, but for the entire military organization. Soldiers who act with integrity are seen as role models and leaders, inspiring trust, respect, and admiration among their peers and superiors. To cultivate integrity, soldiers must be willing to reflect on their values and beliefs and to assess whether their actions are in alignment with these principles. They must also be willing to hold themselves accountable for their actions and to take responsibility for any mistakes or missteps. This requires a strong sense of self-awareness and a commitment to personal growth and development. Soldiers who prioritize integrity also tend to be open-minded and empathetic, seeking to understand and appreciate the perspectives of others while remaining true to their own beliefs and values.

Integrity is a critical quality for soldiers.. It is about doing what is right, even when no one is watching, and remaining true to one's principles and values. Soldiers who prioritize integrity inspire trust, respect, and admiration among their peers and superiors, and help to uphold the values and principles of the military. By cultivating a strong sense of self-awareness, personal accountability, and a commitment to personal growth and development, soldiers can strengthen their integrity and serve as role models for others. These three values are the cornerstone of a soldier's character, and are essential for success both in military service and in life. By upholding the Soldier's Code and living by these values, you can become a soldier, inspiring others to greatness and earning the respect of all those around you .

SECTION I I : SERVICE AND SACRIFICE

The second section of the Soldier's Code is a crucial aspect of being a warrior. As a soldier, it is not just about personal gain or glory, but also about serving a greater cause. The code emphasizes the importance of service and sacrifice, which means being selfless and committed to the greater good, whether that means serving your country, your community, or your family. Service and sacrifice are at the core of what it means to be a soldier. The willingness to make sacrifices and put the needs of others before your own is what sets soldiers apart from others. This selflessness is a hallmark of the warrior spirit, and it is something that every soldier must strive to cultivate.

To truly embrace the ideals of service and sacrifice, soldiers must be willing to go above and beyond what is expected of them. This can involve actively seeking out opportunities to help others, volunteering your time and resources, and being willing to put yourself in harm's way to protect those who cannot protect themselves. But this level of commitment and sacrifice can be emotionally and physically taxing. Soldiers must be prepared for the physical and mental toll that their service may take on them. This can involve developing coping mechanisms to deal with stress and trauma, seeking out support from other soldiers and professionals, and taking care of their own physical and mental health. At the same time, soldiers must be prepared to make difficult choices and face difficult situations. They may be called upon to make sacrifices that are difficult or even impossible to bear. It takes a strong will and a deep sense of commitment to fulfill the second section of the Soldier's Code, but by doing so, soldiers can make a significant and positive impact on the life of others. Living up to the ideals of service and sacrifice requires a deep sense of commitment and a willingness to put the needs of others before your own. By doing so, soldiers can truly live up to the warrior ideals of honor, courage, and selflessness. This is what sets them apart from others and what makes them an essential part of any society. The second section of the Soldier's Code is a reminder that being a soldier is not just a job, but a powerful way of life. It is a calling to something greater than oneself, a commitment to a cause that is bigger than any individual. Soldier, By embracing the ideals of service and sacrifice, you will make a lasting impact on the world around you.

SECTION I I I : BEING A SOLDIER OF POSITIVE INFLUENCE

In this third section of "The Soldier's Code", we are diving deeper into the concept of being a soldier of positive influence. Being a soldier is not just about following a set of codes and making personal sacrifices. It's also about using your power and influence to create a positive impact on the world around you. To do this, it's important to first understand the responsibility that comes with being a soldier of positive influence. This means being accountable for your actions and understanding the impact they have on others. It means taking ownership of your mistakes and making a conscious effort to improve.

Besides personal responsibility, being a soldier of positive influence also requires a certain level of leadership. As a soldier, you can inspire and motivate those around you. You can set an example for others to follow and encourage them to push beyond their limits. Being a leading soldier is not just about giving orders and expecting others to follow blindly. It's about being a role model for those around you and earning their respect through your actions. This means leading by example, being transparent in your communication, and treating others with respect and kindness.As a soldier of positive influence, you also have the power to create change on a larger scale. This can be achieved through community service, volunteering, or even pursuing a career that positively impacts society. By using your skills and talents to benefit others, you can make a real difference in the world. Of course, being a soldier of positive influence is not always easy. It requires hard work, dedication, and a willingness to step outside of your comfort zone. It also requires a deep understanding of your own values and beliefs, and a commitment to upholding them even in the face of . However, the rewards of being a soldier of positive influence are immeasurable. By creating a positive impact on the world around you, you not only improve the lives of those around you, but you also find a deeper sense of purpose and fulfillment in your own life. You become a hero, not just to others, but to yourself as well. Let us embrace our roles as soldiers of positive influence by taking responsibility for our actions, lead by example, and create change in the world. Let us be the heroes we were born to be, and inspire others to do the same. Together, we can make a difference and create a brighter future for ourselves and for generations to come.

PART VI—
OVERCOMING
OBSTACLES

SECTION I : BOUNCING BACK FROM FAILURES

The ability to bounce back from failure is an essential skill for soldiers and civilians alike. Soldiers are trained to operate in high-stress, high-risk situations where failure can have serious consequences. To cope with this pressure, soldiers develop a range of strategies to help them bounce back from failures and setbacks. These same techniques can be applied in real life to help individuals develop greater resilience and overcome challenges.

Acknowledge And Accepte It

The first step in bouncing back from failure is to acknowledge and accept it. Soldiers are trained to take a candid and objective approach to evaluating their performance, recognizing when they fall short of expectations and accepting responsibility for their mistakes. This same approach can be applied in real life by adopting a growth mindset and a willingness to learn from failures. By acknowledging failures and taking ownership of them, individuals can gain valuable insights and develop a better understanding of their strengths and weaknesses.

Developp A Plan Of Improvement

The second step in bouncing back from failure is to develop a plan for improvement. Soldiers are trained to identify the root causes of their failures and to develop strategies to address them. This might involve seeking feedback from colleagues or mentors, taking additional training or education, or simply practicing more. In real life, individuals can apply the same principles by setting specific, measurable, achievable, realistic, and time-bound (SMART) goals to address areas of weakness and improve their performance. By taking an active approach to addressing failures, individuals can develop greater confidence and resilience.

Another technique that soldiers use to bounce back from failure is again to develop a strong support network. Soldiers rely heavily on their fellow soldiers and commanders for guidance, support, and encouragement. This same principle can be applied in real life by building a strong support network of friends, family, colleagues, and mentors who can offer advice, feedback, and encouragement during times of difficulty. By surrounding themselves with positive, supportive people, individuals can build their resilience and overcome setbacks more easily. Soldiers develop a strong sense of purpose and motivation to help them bounce back from failure. Soldiers understand that their work is important and that failure can have serious consequences. This motivates them to work harder and to persist in the face of adversity. In real life, individuals can apply the same principle by developing a strong sense of purpose and motivation for their work. By understanding the importance of what they do and the impact it can have, individuals can find the strength to persist through failures and setbacks and achieve their goals.

SECTION 11 : STAYING STRONG IN THE FACE OF ADVERSITY

When facing difficult circumstances, it's essential to stay mentally strong and resilient. Soldiers are trained to endure and overcome adversity, and there are a few techniques you can use to develop similar traits.

Firstly, It's crucial to have a positive mindset. Focus on the opportunities that may arise from the adversity rather than solely on the challenges. This perspective can help you stay motivated and find creative solutions. Secondly, Develop a strong support system. Soldiers rely on their comrades and superiors for support, and you can benefit from a similar network of friends, family, and colleagues. Surround yourself with people who encourage you, believe in you, and can provide assistance when needed. Third, practice self-care. Make sure to prioritize your physical and mental health. Get enough rest, eat a healthy diet, and exercise regularly. Also, take time to engage in activities that bring you joy and reduce stress, such as reading, spending time in nature, or meditating. Finally, maintain a sense of purpose. Soldiers are motivated by their mission, and you can also stay focused on your goals and aspirations. Having a sense of purpose can give you the strength to endure challenges and keep you motivated even when the going gets tough.By developing a positive mindset, cultivating a strong support system, practicing self-care, and maintaining a sense of purpose, you can stay mentally strong and resilient in the face of adversity, just like a soldier.

SECTION I I I : FUTURE CHALLENGES

This preparation begins long before they face any actual challenges and is an ongoing process throughout their military career. The techniques used by soldiers to prepare for future challenges can also be applied by us in our personal and professional lives.One of the key ways that soldiers prepare for future challenges is by maintaining a strong physical fitness regimen. Soldiers are expected to be in top physical condition to handle the demands of their duties, which often include carrying heavy equipment, navigating difficult terrain, and engaging in combat situations. This physical fitness training not only helps them to meet the physical demands of their duties but also helps them to develop the mental strength and resilience necessary to face challenges head-on.

In addition to physical fitness training, soldiers also receive extensive mental training to prepare for future challenges. This includes learning how to stay calm under pressure, developing mental toughness and resilience, and building problem-solving skills. Soldiers also learn to identify and manage their own emotions and those of others, a critical skill in high-pressure situations. They are trained to stay focused on the mission and to remain calm and composed even in the face of uncertainty and danger. To prepare for future challenges, soldiers also engage in continuous learning and training. They are constantly seeking out new skills and knowledge to stay ahead of the curve and to be ready for any situation that may arise. This includes attending specialized training courses, participating in simulations and exercises, and learning from the experiences of other soldiers. We can use many of the same techniques used by soldiers to prepare for future challenges. We can maintain a strong physical fitness regimen, which not only benefits their physical health but also helps to build mental toughness and resilience. We can also engage in continuous learning and training to stay ahead of the curve and to be ready for any challenges that may come their way, this includes seeking out new skills and knowledge, participating in simulations and exercises, and learning from the experiences of others.

To prepare for future challenges, we can also work on developing their mental and emotional resilience. This includes learning to stay calm and focused under pressure, managing emotions effectively, and building problem-solving skills. By staying focused on our goals and objectives, and developing the mental strength and resilience necessary to overcome obstacles, we can be better prepared for future challenges. Soldiers prepare for future challenges through a combination of physical fitness training, mental toughness and resilience, continuous learning and training, and staying focused on their goals and objectives. By using these techniques,you can be better prepared to face whatever challenges come to you and achieve your goals and objectives.

PART VII - BUILD YOUR STRENGHT

In this chapter, we will explore how soldiers build and maintain their strength, both physical and mental. We will look at the techniques and strategies used by soldiers to develop mental toughness, overcome obstacles, and stay focused on their objectives. We will also examine how we can apply these same techniques in our personal and professional lives to achieve their goals and overcome challenges.

Whether you are looking to improve your physical fitness, develop your mental resilience, or build your problem-solving skills, this chapter will provide you with valuable insights and practical strategies to help you build your strength like a soldier. With the right mindset and training, you too can develop the strength and resilience necessary to overcome any obstacle and achieve your objectives. So let's dive in and explore what it takes to build your strength like a soldier.

SECTION I : THE IMPORTANCE OF SPORT

Sports have always played a significant role in military training, and for good reason. Soldiers are required to be physically and mentally fit, and sports offer a great way to develop both aspects. In fact, many military training programs include sports as an essential component of the overall training regimen.Physical fitness is essential for soldiers, as it directly impacts their ability to perform their duties. Whether it's carrying heavy gear, running long distances, or engaging in combat, soldiers need to be in excellent physical condition. This is where sports come in. Sports provide a fun and engaging way for soldiers to develop their strength, endurance, speed, and agility. Moreover, participating in sports also helps soldiers to build camaraderie and teamwork, both of which are critical in military operations.One of the most significant benefits of sports is that it helps soldiers to develop mental toughness. Mental toughness is the ability to remain focused and motivated under challenging circumstances, and it's a vital trait for soldiers. The stress and pressure of military operations can be overwhelming, but soldiers who have developed mental toughness are better equipped to handle these challenges.Sports provide an excellent opportunity for soldiers to develop mental toughness. Whether it's pushing through physical pain, dealing with setbacks, or staying motivated when the going gets tough, sports teach soldiers the skills they need to develop mental toughness. Moreover, sports provide a safe and controlled environment for soldiers to practice these skills, allowing them to transfer them to real-world situations.Another critical aspect of sports is that they provide soldiers with an opportunity to unwind and relieve stress. Military life can be extremely stressful, and soldiers need to find ways to cope with this stress. Sports provide an excellent outlet for soldiers to blow off steam and relax. Whether it's playing a game of basketball or going for a run, sports offer a healthy and productive way for soldiers to manage stress.Furthermore, sports are also beneficial for soldiers' overall health and wellbeing. Engaging in physical activity regularly can help soldiers to maintain a healthy weight, reduce the risk of chronic diseases, and improve their overall quality of life. It's essential for soldiers to take care of their bodies, and sports provide a fun and engaging way to do so. Sports play a vital role in military training, and soldiers should take advantage of the many benefits they offer. Whether it's developing physical strength, mental toughness, or simply relieving stress, sports provide an excellent way for soldiers to improve their overall health and wellbeing. Moreover, sports help soldiers to build camaraderie and teamwork, critical components of military operations. So, if you want to build your strength like a soldier, start incorporating sports into your training regimen today.

SECTION I I : DEVELOPPING AN EMOTIONNAL TOUGHNESS

As a soldier, you'll face numerous challenges and obstacles that will require you to possess high levels of emotional resilience and fortitude. These skills are essential for handling stressful situations, making tough decisions, and enduring physical and mental hardships while remaining focused on your duty and purpose. However, developing these traits takes effort and time, but with practice, training, and lifestyle choices, it's possible to cultivate them. Emotional resilience is the ability to handle adversity and stress without losing your sense of purpose and direction. To become a resilient soldier, you need to learn how to stay calm and composed under pressure, think on your feet, and adapt to ever-changing situations. You can train your mind to handle stress through deep breathing exercises.

Fortitude is another critical trait that soldiers must possess. It is the strength of mind and spirit to endure hardships and overcome adversity without losing hope or giving up. To develop fortitude, you must have a sense of purpose and meaning in your work, remain committed to your mission and fellow soldiers, and be willing to sacrifice your comfort and safety for the greater good.To cultivate emotional resilience and fortitude, you need to prioritize your physical and mental health. Regular exercise, a balanced diet, and enough sleep are essential to keep your mind and body in top condition. Seeking social support from friends and family, mental health services, can also help you cope with the stresses of military life.Finally, focus on your purpose and goals. Remember the impact you're making on the world and your unit's mission. Align your work with your personal values and goals to create a sense of meaning and purpose. With dedication and effort, you can build the strength and resilience necessary to tackle any challenge that comes your way. As a soldier, these traits will not only help you succeed in your job, but they'll also contribute to your overall well-being.

PART VIII- FACE YOUR FEARS

Surely, you'll face numerous challenges and obstacles that will require you to possess high levels of emotional resilience and fortitude. These skills are essential for handling stressful situations, making tough decisions, and enduring physical and mental hardships while remaining focused on your duty and purpose. However, developing these traits takes effort and time, but with practice, training, and lifestyle choices, it's possible to cultivate them. Emotional resilience is the ability to handle adversity and stress without losing your sense of purpose and direction. To become a resilient soldier, you need to learn how to stay calm and composed under pressure, think on your feet, and adapt to ever-changing situations. You can train your mind to handle stress through deep breathing exercises. Fortitude is another critical trait that soldiers must possess. It is the strength of mind and spirit to endure hardships and overcome adversity without losing hope or giving up. To develop fortitude, you must have a sense of purpose and meaning in your work, remain committed to your mission and fellow soldiers, and be willing to sacrifice your comfort and safety for the greater good.

To cultivate emotional resilience and fortitude, you need

to prioritize your physical and mental health. Regular exercise, a balanced diet, and enough sleep are essential to keep your mind and body in top condition. Seeking social support from friends and family, as well as mental health services, can also help you cope with the stresses of military life.

As a soldier, these traits will not only help you succeed in your job, but they'll also contribute to your overall well-being.

PART IX - APPLYING SOME MILITARY STATEGIES IN REAL LIFE

In the battlefield of life, we face challenges and obstacles that require strategic thinking and planning. In the military, the art of war is the key to success. Let's look at some of the strategies great soldiers used in war and see how we can use them in real life :

George Washington: During the American Revolutionary War, Washington utilized a defensive military strategy. He avoided confrontation with the British army, instead opting to focus on building a strong network of alliances with other European powers and on guerrilla tactics that targeted the enemy's supply lines. This strategy eventually paid off, leading to a victory for the American forces at the Battle of Yorktown in 1781.

Washington's defensive military strategy can also be applied in real-life situations as a valuable lesson in overcoming challenges and obstacles. In personal or professional settings, building strong alliances and networks can provide crucial support in navigating difficult circumstances. By fostering relationships and connections with others who share similar goals or values, one can create a support system that offers guidance, resources, and assistance in times of need. Additionally, Washington's guerrilla tactics can serve as a practical approach in everyday life to tackle obstacles strategically. Being resourceful, creative, and adaptable in problem-solving can help in circumventing challenges and finding alternative solutions. Rather than confronting problems head-on, adopting a more strategic approach by identifying weaknesses in the issue or finding innovative ways to overcome obstacles can lead to successful outcomes. Washington's defensive military strategy and guerrilla tactics are not limited to the battlefield but can also be translated into practical applications in various aspects of life. By focusing on building alliances, networks, and employing strategic problem- solving approaches, one can overcome challenges and achieve success in their personal and professional endeavors, just as Washington's strategy paid off in the eventual victory at the Battle of Yorktown in 1781, which marked a significant turning point in the American Revolutionary War.

General Douglas MacArthur: During World War II, General MacArthur utilized a combination of strategic and tactical military tactics, including the use of amphibious landings, air power, and psychological warfare. He was also known for his "island-hopping" strategy in the Pacific theater, where he bypassed heavily fortified enemy positions and instead captured

less-defended islands to establish airfields and supply bases, allowing for easier access to the Japanese mainland.

General Douglas MacArthur's combined military tactics can be applied in real life to help you overcome problems by encouraging you to take a multifaceted approach to problem- solving. This can involve combining different strategies and techniques to create a more comprehensive and effective solution.

Audie Murphy - Murphy was known for his bravery and determination on the battlefield. He never gave up, even when the odds were against him.
In civilian life, this translates to having a never-say-die attitude and being persistent in the face of obstacles.

Chesty Puller - Puller was a master strategist who always kept his cool under pressure. He was able to think on his feet and come up with creative solutions to complex problems.
It means : being adaptable and able to find solutions to challenges as they arise.

John J. Pershing - Pershing was a great leader who was able to inspire and motivate his troops. He led by example and was always willing to make personal sacrifices for the good of his team.
In real life it's equal to being a great leader who can inspire and motivate others to achieve their goals.

Matthew Ridgway - Ridgway was a master of strategy and tactics. He was able to use his knowledge of the enemy's strengths and weaknesses to gain an

advantage on the battlefield. traduces being able to think strategically and use one's knowledge to gain an advantage over competitors.

Zhang Fei - a general who served under Liu Bei during the Three Kingdoms period and was known for his bravery and ferocity on the battlefield. Zhang Fei was known for his brilliant military strategies, for his ability to read people and situations,his quick thinking and ability to make decisions under pressure, and also for his bravery and willingness to take risks.

In our daily lives, we can apply this by developing our intuition and being observant of situations around us. By doing so, we can make better decisions and avoid potential pitfalls. We can learn to think wisely and make decisions quickly when we are faced with unexpected challenges or situations. This can help us to avoid hesitation and take action to address issues. We can step out of our comfort zones and take calculated risks to achieve our goals. By being courageous and taking bold action, we can accomplish great things that we never thought possible. Soldier, take these lessons from Zhang Fei to heart and apply them in your daily life. Develop your intuition, think quickly, and take calculated risks. With these qualities, you can achieve success in all areas of your life.

PART X- NOW LISTEN TO YOUR MOTIVATIONAL SPEAKER

SECTION I : FORGET ABOUT YOUR PAST FAILURES

I'm sure you've all been there: that moment when you feel like you're stuck in a rut, unable to move forward. Maybe you've made some mistakes in the past, and you feel like they're holding you back. But let me tell you this - your past does not define you. Your failures do not determine your future. So let's begin by forgetting about your past failures and focusing on the present. It's important to understand that everyone makes mistakes. Nobody is perfect, and we all have moments in our lives that we wish we could do over. But the key to moving forward is learning from those mistakes and using them as stepping stones towards success. Remember, every failure is an opportunity to learn and grow. So instead of dwelling on your past mistakes, use them to your advantage, Reflect on what went wrong, identify areas for improvement, and make a plan to move forward. It's also crucial to stop comparing yourself to others. We all have a tendency to compare ourselves to those around us - our friends, our colleagues, even strangers on social media. But the truth is, comparison is the thief of joy. When we focus on what others have accomplished, we lose sight of our own achievements. So instead of measuring your success against others, focus on your own journey. Celebrate your wins, no matter how small, and use them as motivation to keep pushing forward. Remember that you have the power to control your thoughts and emotions. It's easy to get caught up in negative self-talk, telling yourself that you're not good enough or that you'll never succeed. But those thoughts are just that - thoughts. They're not reality. So instead of letting your negative self-talk control you, take charge of your thoughts and turn them into positive affirmations. Tell yourself that you are capable of achieving your goals, and Soldier, see yourself as a winner. Remember, your thoughts and beliefs shape your reality, so make sure they're working for you, not against you. Let go of your past failures, it is essential to your success. Remember that everyone makes mistakes, and that failure is an opportunity to learn and grow. Stop comparing yourself to others and focus on your own journey, celebrating your wins along the way. And most importantly, take control of your thoughts and turn them into positive affirmations. With these tools in your arsenal, you can rise up and become the soldier you were meant to be. So, forget about your pas failures, go out there again and conquer your goals, you will overcome!

SECTION 11 - DON'T COMPROMISE YOUR VALUES

As a soldier, you understand the meaning of sacrifice, commitment, and hard work. You know that success on the battlefield requires bravery, discipline, and a willingness to push past your limits. But what about success in life?

Success is not about compromising your values. True success comes from within, from a deep commitment to your goals and a relentless drive to achieve them. It's about setting your sights on a target and doing whatever it takes to hit it. But what does success look like? For some, it's wealth, power, and fame. For others, it's the satisfaction of a job well done, the love and respect of family and friends, or the knowledge that you've made a difference in the world. Whatever your definition of success, know this: it's within your reach. To achieve success, you must first believe in yourself. You must have faith in your abilities and trust that you have what it takes to overcome any obstacle. You must be willing to work harder than anyone else, to put in the time and effort needed to hone your skills and develop your talents. But don't just work hard; work smart: Learn from your mistakes, study your successes, and never stop learning, yes I say it again, never stop learning. Surround yourself with people who support your goals and inspire you to be your best self. And always remember that success is not a destination; it's a journey. It's a never-ending quest to be the best version of yourself.

So, soldier, I challenge you to rise up and claim your success. Don't let anyone tell you that you can't achieve your dreams or that you have to compromise your values to get ahead. Work hard, and never give up. The world is waiting for you to rise and claim your place in it.

SECTION I I I - YOU ARE A SOLDIER

Ladies and gentlemen, see yourself as a soldier. It's time to rise up and take control of your life, to fight for your dreams and make sacrifices for your future. You are in the midst of an extreme battle, and your success depends on your determination, your focus, and your unwavering commitment to your mission. No matter what your circumstances are, no matter where you come from, no matter what obstacles you face, you have the power within you to rise up again. You are not a victim of your circumstances; you are a warrior, a fighter, a soldier. You have the power to create your own destiny and to live the life you want. But being a soldier is not an easy job. You have to be willing to put in the hard work, to train your mind and body, and to push yourself to your limits. You have to be willing to make sacrifices, to give up things that are holding you back, and to focus on your goals. You have to be willing to fight for what you believe in, and to never give up, no matter how difficult the road may be. You may face disappointments along the way, but don't let them discourage you. Use them as opportunities to learn and grow, and to become stronger and more resilient. Remember that every soldier faces obstacles, but it's how you respond to them that determines your success. So rise up, soldier! Take charge of your life, don't wait for someone else to do it for you. Don't make excuses, build your castle, don't let fear hold you back. You have everything you need to be a winner.

SECTION IV- POSITIVE THOUGHTS AND DREAMS ARE NOT ENOUGH

I want to talk to you about something that is essential to your success: action. You are a member of one of the most disciplined and elite fighting forces in the world and you now know what it takes to be successful. But success is not just about positive thoughts and dreams: It requires action, hard work, and a willingness to face challenges. Positive thinking can help you stay motivated and focused on your goals, but it's not enough. You have to go out there and make it happen. You have to take that first step, even if you're afraid. You have to push yourself out of your comfort zone and do things that are difficult and uncomfortable. Success also requires hard work. You can day in and day out become the best soldier you can be. But you can't just coast through life and expect to achieve your goals. You have to put in the time and effort to make things happen. You have to be willing to sacrifice short-term pleasures for long-term gains.

The other requirement of success is a willingness to face challenges. As a soldier, you know that the path to victory is often paved with obstacles. You can't just give up when things get tough. You have to be willing to fight through adversity and keep pushing forward. You have to be willing to take risks and make mistakes, knowing that failure is just a temporary setback on the road to success. So, soldier, if you want to be successful, you have to be willing to take action, work hard, and face any challenges. You have to be willing to do whatever it takes to make your dreams come true. Remember, success is not just about positive thoughts and dreams, it's about taking action, working hard, and never giving up. I know that you have the potential to achieve greatness,you have what it takes to be successful. But it's up to you to make it happen, go out there and do what it takes to make your dreams a reality. Rise up and be the best soldier you can be.

SECTION V- CHOOSE FIGHT, CHOOSE WAR, CHOOSE YOUR BATTLEFIELD

Soldier, It's time to wake up and realize that life is a battlefield, and you are the warrior. You have to choose your battles, pick up your weapons, and fight with all your might. If you are not ready to fight, then you will never win the war. Life is full of challenges, obstacles, and difficulties, some people run away from them, while others face them head-on. The difference between a winner and a loser is the courage to fight, the boldness of a lion: The willingness to take on challenges and overcome them. The determination to never give up, no matter how hard the battle gets. My friend, are you ready to fight? Are you ready to face your fears, your doubts, your weaknesses, and your failures? Are you ready to step onto the battlefield and give it your all? Because if you are, then you will emerge victorious.Remember, soldiers overcome, but warriors never quit. You must have these traits in your spirit, my friend. You have to be the one who never gives up, who never backs down, who never surrenders. You have to be the one who keeps fighting, even when the battle seems lost.The world needs warriors like you, people who are willing to fight for what they believe in, for what they love, for what they want to achieve. People who are not afraid of the challenges, but embrace them. People who are not afraid to fail, but use their failures as stepping stones to success. So, my friend, choose your battles wisely. Choose the ones that matter to you, the ones that align with your values, your passions, and your dreams.Choose the ones that will make you grow, that will make you stronger, that will make you a better person. And when you choose your battles, choose your weapons carefully. Your weapons are your skills, your knowledge, your attitude, and your mindset. Sharpen them, polish them, and make them the best they can be. Use them wisely, strategically, and effectively.

The greatest battlefield is not out there, but inside of you. It's in your mind, in your heart, in your soul. It's the battle between your fears and your dreams, your doubts and your confidence, your weaknesses and your strengths. It's the battle that will define who you are and what you can become.So, my friend, choose fight, choose war, choose the battlefield. And do it with all your heart, all your soul, and all your mind. And never forget that you are a warrior, a fighter, a winner. You deserve to be successful, and you will be. Just believe in yourself and keep fighting.

SECTION VI- THERE ARE NO EXCUSES IN WAR ZONE

Soldier, great leaders come in all shapes and sizes. They are found on the battlefield, in the boardroom, and on the sports field. They are men and women who have overcome great adversity, who have fought hard and persevered in the face of challenges. They are individuals who have embodied the spirit of the lion, and have risen up to become legends in their own time.

Let's Talk Of:

Michael Jordan, widely regarded as one of the greatest basketball players of all time, faced challenges and setbacks throughout his career. He was cut from his high school basketball team, faced tough competition in the NBA, and experienced failures in playoff games. But Jordan's unrelenting determination, work ethic, and competitive spirit helped him overcome these obstacles and achieve unparalleled success in the world of basketball.

Mike Tyson, a former professional boxer, faced numerous challenges and setbacks both inside and outside the boxing ring. He battled personal demons, legal issues, and controversies throughout his career. But Tyson's relentless fighting spirit, his determination to bounce back from defeats, and his resilience in the face of adversity made him one of the most feared and respected boxers in the history of the sport.

Samuel Eto'o: The new president of "FECAFOOT" is a real soldier. He was born in Cameroon and grew up in poverty, but he never let his circumstances define him. Instead, he fought hard and honed his skills as a soccer player, becoming one of the greatest African players of all time. He won multiple championships, including three UEFA Champions League titles, and was a four-time African Player of the Year.

Francis Ngannou, the Cameroonian-born, mixed martial artist, is another example of a true soldier who has overcome tremendous adversity. Ngannou faced extreme poverty and hardships in his early life, and he was forced to leave his home in search of a better future. He worked odd jobs to survive, and it was during this time that he discovered his talent for fighting. Ngannou eventually found his way to France and pursued a career in mixed martial arts. Despite facing numerous challenges and setbacks, Ngannou never lost sight of his goal. He trained tirelessly, honing his skills and improving his technique. He faced defeats and setbacks in his early fights, but he refused to give up. Instead, he learned from his mistakes and continued to push forward, displaying the unwavering determination and resilience of a true soldier. In 2018, Ngannou's hard work and perseverance paid off when he won the UFC Heavyweight Championship, becoming the first African-born fighter to hold the title. His incredible journey from poverty to championship glory is a testament to his unbreakable spirit and warrior mindset. Ngannou's story is a reminder that there are no excuses in the war zone of life. Despite the challenges we face, we must keep pushing forward, never giving up on our dreams and aspirations.

Ngannou's success in the octagon also extends beyond his fighting skills. He has become an inspiration to many, not just for his athletic achievements, but for his humble and gracious attitude. He has used his platform to advocate for social issues, including raising awareness about the struggles of his homeland in Africa. Ngannou's story serves as a powerful example of how a true soldier uses his success to make a positive impact on the world.

Conor McGregor, a professional mixed martial artist, faced challenges and setbacks in his early career. He was a relatively unknown fighter from Ireland who faced skepticism and doubts from the MMA community. However, McGregor's self-belief, confidence, and unshakable determination led him to become, a two-division UFC champion, a true soldier, one of the most recognizable and successful fighters in the world.

Tiger Woods: In the early 2000s, professional golfer Tiger Woods was at the top of his game. He had won numerous championships, including 14 major titles, and was considered one of the greatest golfers of all time. Unfortunately, in 2009, Woods' career and personal life took a hit when news broke of his infidelity and subsequent divorce. He took a break from golf to address his personal issues and did not return to competitive play for several months. When he did return, Woods struggled with injuries and inconsistent play, and many believed his career was over. But Woods refused to give up. He continued to work hard on his game, and in 2018, he achieved a stunning comeback by winning the Tour Championship, his first victory in five years. Woods' perseverance and determination paid off when, in 2019, he won his fifth Masters Tournament, one of the most prestigious events in golf. His comeback was nothing short of inspiring, and it showed that even the greatest of athletes can face setbacks but still rise up again to achieve greatness. based upon this text add and explain the fact that wood demonstrated he has the spirit of a soldier, of a warrior. Woods faced a personal and professional crisis that could have destroyed him. But he didn't let it defeat him. Like a soldier in battle, he took a step back to address his personal issues and regain his strength. He faced his injuries and inconsistent play head-on, refusing to give up on his mission. Through hard work and determination, Woods emerged victorious once again. He proved that setbacks are not the end of the road but merely a detour on the path to greatness. And just like a soldier who has been knocked down, he rose up stronger than ever before. But Woods' story is not just about golf. It's a lesson in resilience for all of us. Life is full of challenges that test us, and it's up to us to choose how we respond. We can either give up or rise up like true warriors. So, rise up, soldier! Don't let setbacks define you. You are stronger than you know, and you have the unbreakable spirit of a warrior within you. No matter what obstacles you face, remember that you have the power to overcome them. It won't be easy, but it will be worth it. Every time you face a setback, think of Woods and his never-give- up attitude. Remember that you too can rise up and overcome anything that comes your way. It's time to show the world what you're made of, soldier. In the words of Woods himself, 'If you're not failing, you're not trying hard enough.

Lionel Messi and Cristiano Ronaldo: two soccer players who have dominated the sport for over a decade. They have broken records, won countless awards, and have shown a level of dedication and commitment to their craft that is truly inspiring.

Barack Obama: was the first African American President of the United States, and he faced intense opposition and criticism throughout his presidency. But he never wavered in his commitment to his ideals, and he worked tirelessly to improve the lives of millions of Americans.

Arnold Schwarzenegger, a bodybuilder, actor, and politician, faced challenges as an immigrant to the United States and initially struggled with English language and cultural barriers. He faced criticism and setbacks in his early bodybuilding career, but he remained committed to his goals and eventually became a seven- time Mr. Olympia champion and one of the most successful action movie stars of all time. Schwarzenegger then transitioned into a successful political career, serving as the Governor of california.

Jason Statham: known for his roles as an action hero in movies, was a member of Britain's National Diving Squad before he became an actor. He faced challenges and setbacks, but he never gave up on his dream of becoming an actor. He honed his skills, worked hard, and persevered, eventually becoming a successful actor known for his tough and resilient characters on-screen.

Sylvester Stallone, best known for his role as Rocky Balboa in the Rocky movie series, he faced rejection and setbacks early in his acting career. He was told he wasn't the right fit for leading roles due to his speech impediment and unconventional looks. But Stallone refused to give up on his dream of becoming an actor and wrote the script for Rocky, a story about an underdog fighter who overcomes adversity. Despite facing multiple rejections, Stallone fought for his vision and eventually secured the lead role in the movie. Rocky became a blockbuster success and launched Stallone's career as a Hollywood action star.

Jackie Chan, a martial artist, actor, and stuntman, has faced numerous challenges and injuries throughout his career due to his physically demanding roles. He has broken bones, dislocated joints, and suffered other injuries while performing his own stunts. But Chan's unwavering dedication to his craft and his willingness to push through challenges have made him one of the most respected and successful martial artists and actors in the world. These people are great examples, they have all overcome adversity and have shown the fighting spirit of a soldier. They have faced challenges, setbacks, and obstacles, but they never gave up. They fought hard, stayed committed to their goals, and emerged as legends in their respective fields.

SECTION VII- NEVER GIVE UP

I want you to listen to these words very carefully, for they carry the key to your success : warriors never give up, soldiers never quit. When you find yourself in the heat of battle, whether it be a physical or mental one, you must never surrender. You are a fighter, a champion, and you have the power and ability in you to overcome any obstacle that comes your way. So, stand tall and keep fighting. Believe in yourself and your abilities, for they are far greater than you can imagine. You have a mission to fulfill, a purpose to serve, and you cannot afford to give up now. You cannot let your guard down, even for a moment. You must keep pushing forward, no matter how hard it gets.In life, we face many battles. Some of these battles are physical, such as when we are competing in sports or fighting in a war. But most battles we face are mental. We battle with ourselves, with our doubts and fears. We battle with the people around us, with their negative opinions and criticisms. And we battle with the world itself, with its challenges and obstacles.But no matter what battle you are facing, remember this: you are a warrior. You were born to fight. You were born to win. So don't give up. Don't quit. Don't let anyone or anything break you down.When you are in a battle, you need to be prepared. You need to be strong, both physically and mentally. You need to have a clear focus, a strong will, and an unshakable determination. You need to know your strengths and weaknesses, and use them to your advantage. And most importantly, you need to have faith in yourself, in your abilities, and in your purpose. But being a warrior is not just about being prepared. It's also about being fearless. It's about taking risks, even when you are scared. It's about being bold and daring, and never backing down from a challenge.So my friend, I want you to be a warrior. I want you to be fearless. I want you to face your battles with confidence and strength. I want you to be the kind of person who never gives up, no matter how hard it gets. When you face those battles, let people speechless, show them what you are made of. I want you to be so strong, so determined, so unstoppable, because you are a strong soldier. A good fighter can win the battle but good soldier they dominate battles. They don't just survive; they thrive. They don't just achieve success; they leave a lasting legacy. I challenge you today, to be an unforgettable soldier, I challenge you to never quit no matter how hard the war gets. Your rewards and records must leave others speechless.

SECTION VIII : MAKE MAMA PROUD

Soldier ! I want to talk to you about something that is near and dear to all of our hearts: making Mama proud. Now, Mama may mean different things to different people. She could be your actual mother, your grandmother, your auntie, your mentor, or someone who has simply been there for you through thick and thin. But one thing is certain: Mama wants you to succeed. Mama wants you to be the best version of yourself, to achieve your dreams, and to make a difference in the world. So how do we make Mama proud? We do it by rising up. We do it by standing tall and taking charge of our lives. We do it by fighting for what we believe in, sacrificing our present for a better future, and never giving up on our goals. I know it's not easy. Life can be tough, and sometimes it feels like the odds are stacked against us. But let me tell you something: you are stronger than you think. You have the power within you to overcome any obstacle, to persevere through any hardship, and to   achieve any goal   you   set your mind to. But it all starts with a choice. You have to choose to rise up. You have to choose to take charge of your life. You have to choose to make Mama proud. How do you do that? You do it by setting goals and working tirelessly to achieve them. You do it by staying focused and disciplined, even when the going gets tough. You do it by surrounding yourself with positive people who believe in you and support your dreams.

And most importantly, you do it by never giving up.

There will be setbacks and failures along the way, but you can't let them defeat you. You have to pick yourself up, dust yourself off, and keep pushing forward. Remember, soldier: making Mama proud isn't just about achieving your own goals. It's also about giving back to your community, your country, and the world at large. It's about using your talents and abilities to make a positive impact on the world. I challenge you soldier, to rise up, to take charge of your life, to fight for your dreams and never give up, to make Mama proud. Because when you do, you're not just making Mama proud - you're making yourself proud, and you're making the world a better place.

SECTION IX : YOU WILL WIN

Soldier, as you read this, know that you are not here by chance or coincidence. You are part of an elite team, carefully selected and trained to achieve greatness. You have undergone rigorous lessons and preparation to become the best of the best, and now is the time to put that training to use. But being born to win is just the beginning. To truly succeed, you must believe in your own abilities, have unwavering confidence in yourselves, and be committed to the mindset of a winner. In this team of winners, there is no room for doubt or hesitation. You must have the unwavering conviction that you are capable of accomplishing anything you set your minds to. You must be resilient in the face of challenges, never wavering in your determination to overcome any obstacles that come your way. As soldiers, you are not just physically strong, but also mentally tough. You have the courage to face adversity head-on and the resilience to keep pushing forward, no matter how tough the battle may be. But remember, you are not alone. You are part of a team that is united in mindset and purpose. You have comrades who share the same goals and are committed to supporting each other. In this team, we fight together, we win together. We have each other's backs, and we never leave a fallen comrade behind. We are bound by a common purpose, and we will overcome any challenges that come our way as a team. Remember that you are a part of a team of winners, you have the strength within you to keep going, the courage to persevere, and the determination to overcome any obstacles. You will not give up, and you will not surrender. You will rise above every challenge, knowing that you are capable of greatness. Soldier, from this moment on, move forward with your head held high, knowing that you are a part of a team that is destined for success. Your spirit is unbreakable, your resolve unwavering, and your heart full of determination. You were born to win, and nothing will stand in your way. Together, we will achieve unbelievable things, and we will show the world what it truly means to be a winner. So, as the war has begun, rise up, soldier! Let us go out there and show the world what we are made of. Yes, let us embody the spirit of a winner in everything we do, and let us leave our mark in history as a team that never backed down, never gave up, and emerged victorious against all odds. Soldier, you are winner, and together, we will conquer every challenge that comes our way. Onward to victory!

SECTION X MARCH FORWARD WITH COURAGE

As you march forward towards your goals, remember that courage is not just a virtue, but your most powerful weapon. It takes immense courage to choose to face challenges head-on, to persevere in the face of adversity, and to continue pushing forward even when the path seems difficult. Just like a soldier on the battlefield, courage is not just about bravery, but also about unwavering determination and resilience. It's about choosing to fight rather than flee, and to keep going despite the obstacles that may come your way. It's about being willing to take risks and step out of your comfort zone in pursuit of your dreams. As you face challenges and obstacles along your journey towards success, remember to let your actions speak louder than your words. Be the example that inspires and leaves others speechless. Show others what true courage looks like by your unwavering commitment to your goals, your refusal to back down, and your relentless pursuit of excellence. But remember, you are not alone in this journey. You are part of a larger community of warriors who have faced similar challenges and have overcome them. Just like in the "Great Motivational Book Ever: Rise Up Soldier," which speaks of strength, perseverance, and determination, let those words guide you in your moments of doubt or difficulty. Keep reminding yourself that you have the strength and tenacity to overcome any obstacle that comes your way. Moreover, take a moment to reflect on those who have supported you throughout your journey. Whether it's your parents, siblings, spouse, children, or friends, acknowledge their love and support as a source of motivation. Let their belief in you fuel your courage and determination to keep pushing forward, even when the going gets tough. As you march forward with courage towards your goals, remember that success is not just about achieving personal greatness, but also about making those who love you proud. Your courage and determination will not only benefit you, but also inspire and impact those around you. Your journey towards success can serve as a beacon of hope and encouragement for others who may be facing their own challenges. Finally, never forget that the greatest victory is the one you achieve over yourself. It's about conquering your limitations. It's about pushing past your comfort zone and embracing the unknown. It's about realizing your own potential and constantly striving to become the best version of yourself. So, as you continue on your journey towards success, march forward with courage, soldier. Embrace the challenges, persevere through the obstacles, and keep pushing forward with unwavering determination. With the love and support of those who believe in you, you are capable of achieving anything you set your mind to. Remember, faith is your most valuable weapon, and you have it within you to achieve greatness. Keep marching forward with courage, and let your journey be a testament to the warrior within you.

THE END

The book "Best Motivational Book Ever: Rise Up Soldier" has been a beacon of inspiration, showing us that we possess an inherent power within ourselves to overcome any obstacle that comes our way. Through its pages, you have been reminded that rising up is not a one-time event, but rather a continuous process that requires unwavering determination and perseverance. The author of the book has delved into the depths of human resilience, highlighting the importance of facing our fears and doubts head-on. It emphasizes the need to push ourselves beyond our comfort zones and to never give up on our dreams, no matter how daunting the challenges may seem. In a world that often throws curveballs at us, the book reminds us that we have the capacity to rise above and conquer any adversity that comes our way. Drawing on the metaphor of a soldier, the book encourages us to march forward with courage and conviction. Just like soldiers on the battlefield, we must be resilient and tenacious in our pursuit of success. We must not shy away from taking risks or facing setbacks, but rather embrace them as opportunities for growth and learning. The book instills in us the belief that we are capable of achieving greatness if we set our minds to it and persevere with unwavering determination. Furthermore, the book emphasizes the importance of self-belief. It highlights that in order to rise up, we must first believe in ourselves and our capabilities. Our mindset plays a crucial role in our journey towards success. With the right attitude and a positive outlook, we can overcome any obstacle and achieve our goals. The book encourages us to cultivate a mindset of resilience, optimism, and self-confidence.The message of the book is clear - no matter where we are in life, it is never too late to rise up and pursue our dreams. It reminds us that we are not defined by our past failures or limitations, but rather by our ability to rise above them and strive for excellence. It encourages us to embrace challenges as opportunities for growth and to push ourselves beyond our perceived limitations.

"Best Motivational Book Ever: Rise Up Soldier" serves as a powerful reminder that we are capable of overcoming any obstacle and achieving our goals. It inspires you to be resilient, courageous, and determined in your pursuit of success. Through its pages, you are reminded that you possess the power within you to rise up, face challenges, and march forward towards victory. From now on : make that first step towards your brighter future, armed with the wisdom and motivation imparted by this exceptional book and continue to rise up every single day.

ABOUT THE AUTHOR

Atty Bayeba Arnaud Didace

ATTY BAYEBA Arnaud Didace is a dynamic businessman, inspirational writer and speaker, researcher, and financial manager. His passion for empowering individuals to achieve their goals has led him to become a highly sought-after motivational speaker. In addition to his professional achievements, he is always seeking to inspire others to embrace their full potential, take action, build and achieve their dreams.

Contact the author at : arnauddidace365@outlook.com